My Mediterranean Diet Plan

Quick, Easy & Tasty Mediterranean Recipes to Lose Weight With Taste

Jenna Violet

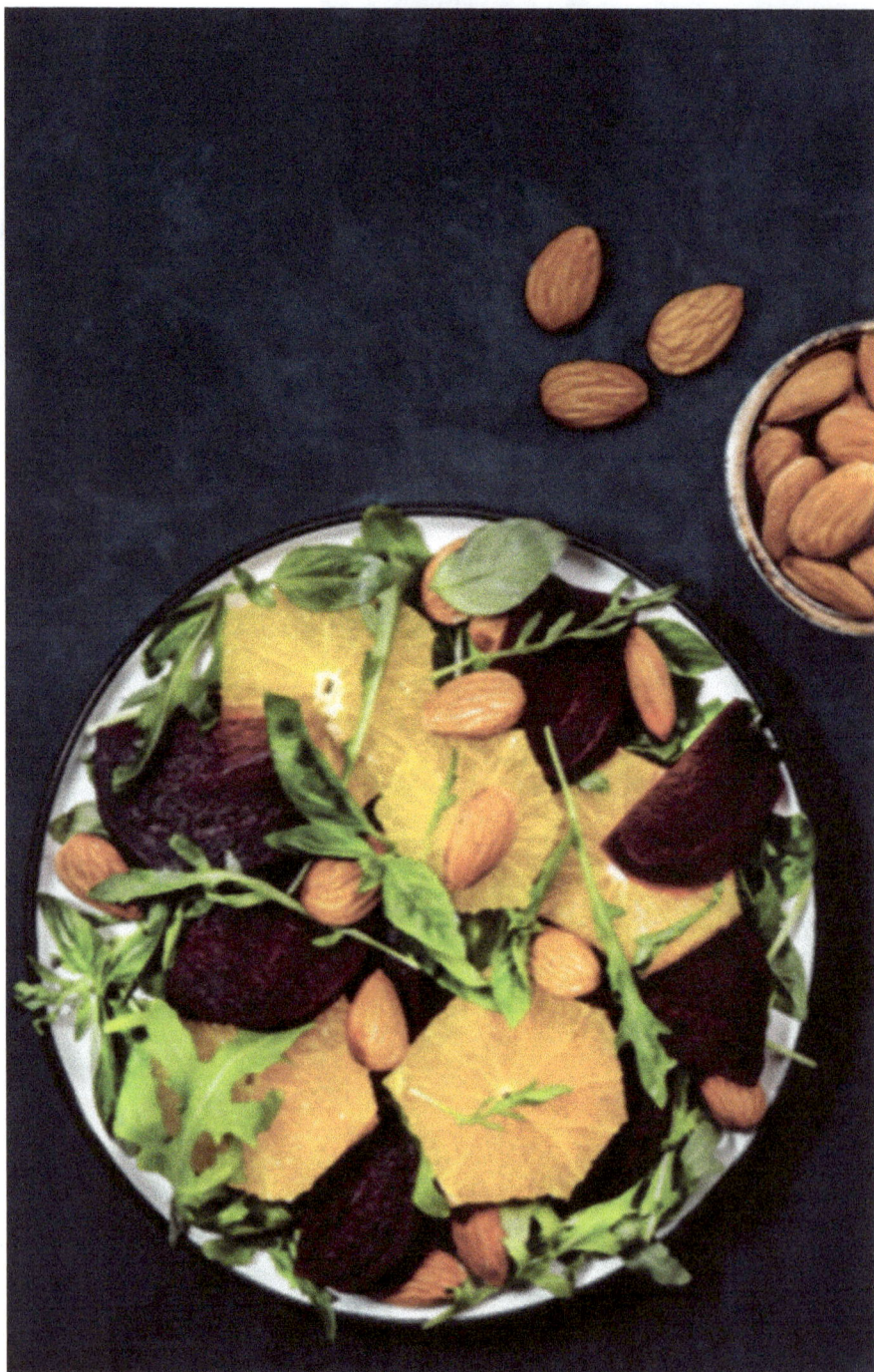

Table of Contents

Spinach and mozzarella egg bake

Ingredients

- 8 eggs, beaten
- 5 oz. of organic fresh spinach
- salt and fresh ground black pepper
- 2 teaspoon of olive oil
- 1 teaspoon of spike seasoning
- 1 ½ cups of grated mozzarella cheese
- 1/3 cup of thinly sliced green onions

Directions

- Preheat your oven to 375°F.
- Spray a glass casserole dish with olive oil.
- Then, heat the olive oil in a large frying pan.
- Add spinach all at once, and stir just until the spinach is wilted.
- Transfer spinach to the casserole dish, spreading it around to cover the dish bottom.
- Layer the grated cheese and sliced onions on top of the spinach.
- Beat the eggs with spike seasoning, and salt and fresh ground pepper

- Pour the egg mixture over the spinach combination

- Then, let bake for 35 minutes or until the mixture is completely set.

- Let cool for 5 minutes.

- Serve and enjoy when hot.

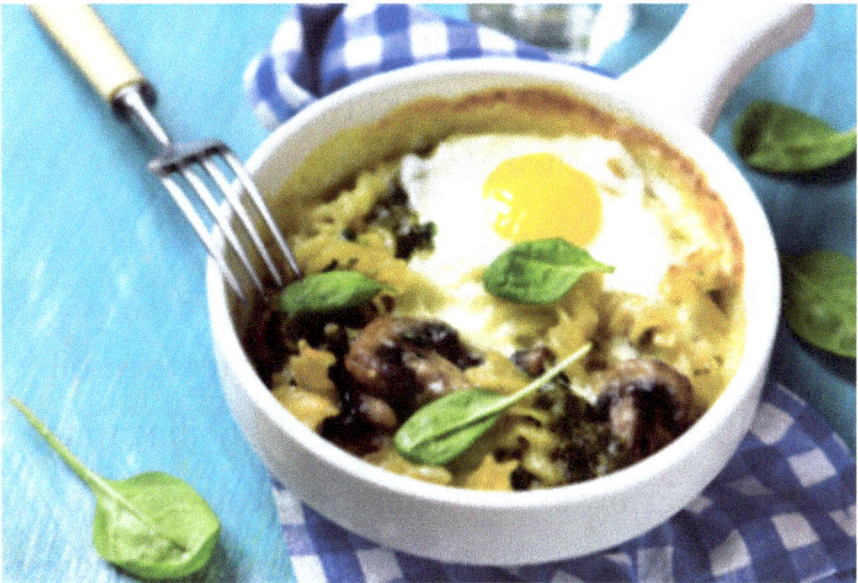

Broccoli, ham, and mozzarella baked with eggs

Ingredients

- 1 teaspoon of spike seasoning
- 10 eggs, beaten well
- 6 cups of chopped broccoli pieces
- 1/3 cup of thinly sliced green onion
- 2 cups of diced ham
- Fresh-ground black pepper
- 1 cup of grated Mozzarella

Directions

- Firstly, heat your oven ready to 375°F.
- Bring a medium-sized pot of water to a boil.
- Cook the broccoli briefly in the boiling water.
- Drain any excess water into a colander.
- Layer broccoli, ham, Mozzarella, and green onions in casserole dish.
- Season with spike seasoning and fresh-ground black pepper.
- Then pour beaten egg over.

- Stir the mixture until all the ingredients are coated with egg.
- Let bake until all the mixture is set in 45 minutes.
- Serve and enjoy with sour cream.

Vegan hummus toasted sandwich

Ingredients

- 3 tablespoons of hummus
- 2 slices of bread
- 1 ripe avocado, thinly sliced
- Salt and pepper
- 1 tablespoon of olive oil
- A handful of rocket
- 4 thin slices of butternut
- ¼ teaspoon of smoked paprika

Directions

- Begin by toasting the slices of bread in a toaster.
- Then, heat 1 tablespoon of the olive oil in a frying pan
- Once hot, add the butternut squash together with the smoked paprika and salt and pepper
- Fry until the squash is soft and golden brown on both sides in 10 minutes or so.
- Spread the hummus on one of the pieces of toasted bread, top with the squash, slices of

avocado, and handful of rocket, combine together.

- Serve and enjoy with lemon squeezed over the avocado.

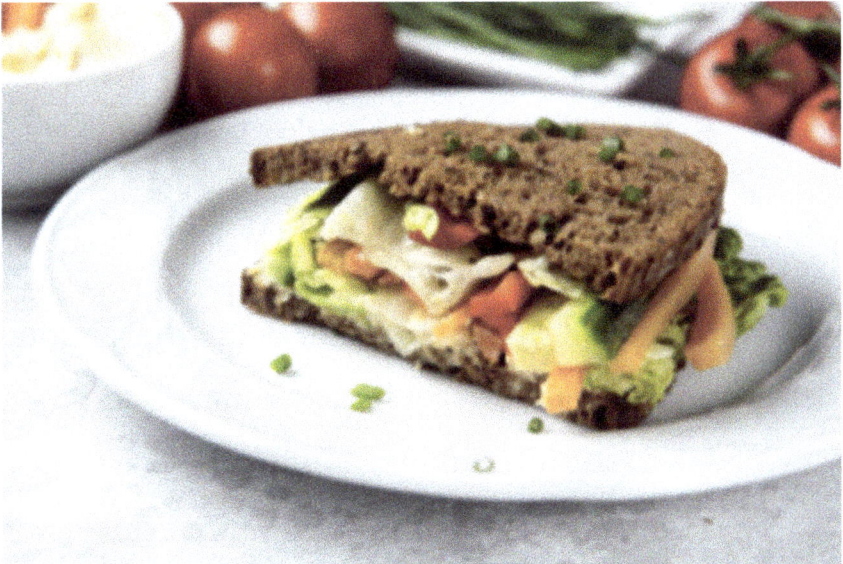

Honey almond ricotta spread with fruit

Ingredients

- Hearty whole grain toast
- Sliced peaches
- 1 cup of whole milk ricotta
- ½ cup of almonds
- ¼ teaspoon of almond extract
- Zest from an orange
- Extra fisher sliced almonds
- 1 teaspoons of honey

Directions

- Combine ricotta together with the almonds and almond extract in a medium sized mixing bowl, stir to combine.
- Transfer to a serving bowl and sprinkle with additional sliced almonds.
- Drizzle with a teaspoon of honey.
- Toast, and spread 1 tablespoon of ricotta on each slice of bread.
- Top with sliced peaches, sliced almonds and honey.
- Serve and enjoy.

Baked eggs with avocado and feta

Ingredients

- Salt and fresh-ground black pepper
- 2 teaspoons of crumbled Feta Cheese
- 1 avocado
- 4 eggs
- Olive oil

Directions

- Break eggs into individual ramekins and let the eggs and avocado come to room temperature.
- Set your oven ready to 400°F.
- Place the gratin dishes on a baking sheet and heat them in the oven for 10 minutes.
- Remove gratin dishes from the oven and spray with olive oil.
- Arrange the sliced avocados in each dish, then, break 2 eggs into each dish.
- Sprinkle with crumbled Feta.
- Then, season with salt and fresh-ground black pepper.

- Let bake until the whites are set and the egg yolks are done to your choice.
- Serve and enjoy.

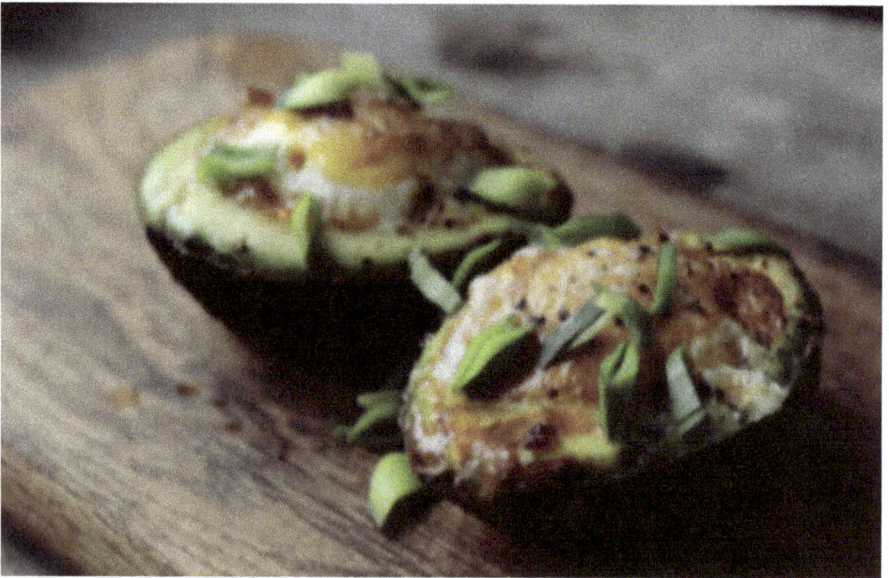

Mediterranean sheet pan salmon

The Mediterranean sheet pan salmon recipe is inspired by Mediterranean ingredients packed with omega 3s. additionally, it features variety of great vegetables for a perfect healthy meal.

Ingredients

- kosher salt and fresh cracked pepper
- 2 small lemons thinly sliced
- ½ cup pitted assorted olives
- Fresh herbs
- 2 tablespoon of salted butter cut in small chunks
- Large whole salmon filet
- 2 cups cherry tomatoes halved
- A few marinated sweet or hot peppers
- 2 teaspoons of capers
- ¼ red onion thinly sliced, rings separated
- 4 tablespoon of extra virgin olive oil

Directions

- Start by preheating your oven ready to 425°F.

- Line a baking sheet with parchment paper and lay out your fish.
- Organize the lemon slices on and around the fish, along with the olives, tomatoes, peppers, capers, and onions.
- Drizzle olive oil all over.
- Sprinkle with salt and pepper.
- Dot with chunks of butter.
- Let bake for 30 minutes, or until the fish is done through.
- Lastly, garnish with fresh herbs.
- Serve and enjoy.

Creamy tomato and roasted veggie risotto

Ingredients

- A small bunch of fresh basil, torn
- Salt and pepper, to taste
- 300g of cherry tomatoes
- 2 red peppers
- 1 large courgette, zucchini
- A generous pinch of salt and pepper
- Vegan parmesan
- 1 tablespoon of olive oil
- 1 large red onion, diced
- 3 garlic cloves, minced
- 1 tablespoon of olive oil
- 225g of risotto rice
- 1 tablespoon of balsamic vinegar
- 250ml of passata
- 250ml of vegetable stock
- 6 sun-dried tomatoes

Directions

- Preheat the oven to 350°F.
- Add the olive oil to a roasting tin.

- Chop and spread vegetables out in the tin.
- Add salt and pepper, shake to coat.
- Let roast for 30 minutes.
- Add olive oil to a shallow casserole dish over a low-medium heat.
- Sauté the onion briefly, then add the minced garlic, cook further for another minute.
- Stir in the rice with the vinegar, stir to coat with the olive oil.
- Pour in the passata and vegetable stock, ½ cup at a time, alternating between the two.
- Let each amount be absorbed by the rice before adding the next.
- After 20 minutes, add in the sundried tomatoes together with the roasted vegetables.
- Remove from the heat and stir in the basil, salt and pepper and vegan cheese.
- Serve and enjoy immediately.

Yogurt tahini Mediterranean carrot salad

Ingredients

- 1/3 cup of crumbled feta
- 2 tablespoons of tahini
- ½ cup of chopped parsley
- 2 tablespoons of water
- Salt and pepper to taste
- ¼ cup of plain Greek yogurt
- 1 tablespoon of lime juice
- ½ tablespoon of honey
- Black sesame seeds for garnish
- 2 large carrots
- 15 ounces can of chickpeas, drained and rinse
- ½ cup of royal raisins

Directions

- Place tahini in a food processor with bit of water. Process until smooth.
- Add the yogurt together with lime juice and honey, process again until smooth.

- Using a spiralizer on blade or a julienne peeler make noodles from the carrots and trim into manageable sizes.
- Place the carrot noodles in a large bowl.
- Add the chickpeas together with the raisins, parsley and feta.
- Add the dressing and toss until well combined.
- Season with salt and pepper to taste.
- Garnish with black sesame seeds.
- Serve and enjoy.

Greek style lemon roasted potatoes

Ingredients

- 1 tablespoon of dried oregano
- 5 lb. Bag of potatoes peeled and quartered
- ¼ cup of olive oil
- 1 lemon juiced
- 1 tablespoon of garlic powder
- 2 teaspoon of salt
- 1 teaspoon of freshly ground pepper

Directions

- Firstly, preheat your oven ready to 400°F.
- Spray a dish with cooking spray and set aside.
- Spread quartered potatoes into an even layer in the pan.
- Juice 1 lemon and pour over the potatoes.
- Cut the lemon peel into small chunks and also add to the pan.
- Add olive oil together with the salt and pepper, oregano, and garlic powder to the pan.
- Stir with a large spoon to combine.

- Let bake for 45 minutes, turning twice with a metal spatula.

- Taste a bite and adjust the seasoning.

- Garnish with parsley, serve and enjoy.

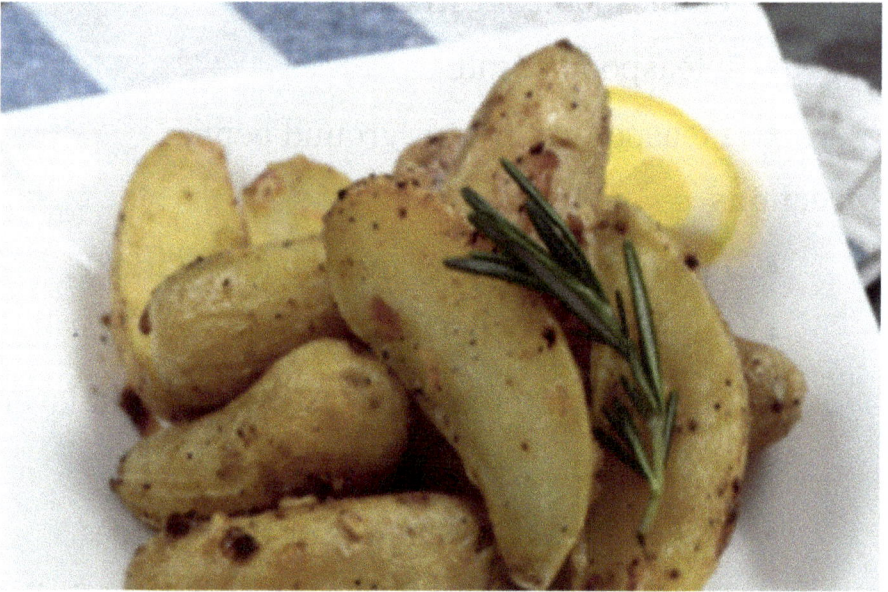

Honey lemon ricotta breakfast toast with figs and pistachios

Ingredients

- 2 tablespoons of pistachio pieces
- 2 slices of whole grain
- 4 figs, sliced
- ¼ cup of low fat ricotta
- 1 teaspoon of lemon zest
- ½ fresh lemon, juiced
- ½ tablespoon of honey

Directions

- Toast bread in toaster.
- Then, whip ricotta together with the lemon juice and honey until smooth and creamy.
- Spread ricotta moisture evenly over each piece of toast.
- Top with sliced figs.
- Sprinkle each piece with pistachio pieces and lemon zest.
- Serve and enjoy.

Breakfast tabbouleh

Ingredients

- ½ cup of bulgur
- 4 tablespoons of olive oil
- 8 large eggs
- 2 cups of fresh Italian flat-leaf parsley, chopped
- ½ pint of grape or cherry tomatoes, diced
- 8 pita wedges
- 1 tablespoon of white vinegar
- ½ cucumber, diced
- Zest and juice of ½ medium lemon
- 1 teaspoon of coarse salt
- ½ teaspoon of ground black pepper

Directions

- Bring 1 cup of water to a boil.
- Then, add bulgur, let cook at a simmer rate for 12 minutes or until water has absorbed, stirring regularly.
- Let cool briefly, then place in an airtight container in the refrigerator until completely cooled.

- In a medium mixing bowl, stir together cooled bulgur, cucumber, lemon juice, olive oil, parsley, tomatoes, salt and pepper.
- Taste, and adjust seasoning accordingly. Place in the refrigerator.
- Bring a large pot of salted water to a simmer.
- Add vinegar and stir to combine.
- Break eggs into the simmering water, one at a time.
- Carefully scoop each egg with a slotted spoon.
- Let eggs cook 3 minutes, until white is set.
- Remove and lay the eggs on a paper towel to dry.
- Scoop tabbouleh and poached eggs on plates.
- Serve and enjoy with pita wedges.

Scrambled eggs in a caramelized onions and paprika

Ingredients

- 2 teaspoons of mixed herb
- 3 tablespoons of Parsley
- 4 Eggs
- 2 tablespoons of olive oil
- 1 medium onion, sliced
- Salt to taste
- 2 teaspoons of chili garlic oil
- 1 large diced tomato
- 1 tablespoon of Feta cheese
- 1 small cube of capsicum
- 3 cloves of garlic, minced
- 2 teaspoons of smoked paprika
- ½ tablespoon of Turmeric

Directions

- Begin by heating the olive oil over medium heat and caramelize onion till they turn dark in 15 minutes.

- Place in the capsicum together with the chili garlic oil. Mix well.
- Add the tomatoes together with the turmeric, garlic, and the mixed herbs.
- Let cook with a tablespoon of water for 5 minutes or so.
- Then, add the paprika.
- Whisk the eggs till frothy.
- Add the eggs, leave to set in 30 seconds.
- Then gently mix it all together.
- Add salt and adjust accordingly to your taste.
- Remove from heat once eggs are set well.
- Lastly, garnish with parsley and feta.
- Serve and enjoy.

Spicy sweet potato hummus

Ingredients

- 1 ½ teaspoon of cayenne pepper
- 2 medium sweet potatoes
- ½ teaspoon of smoked paprika
- 3 tablespoons of olive oil
- ¼ teaspoon of cumin
- 2 cups of cooked chickpeas
- 3 cloves garlic, peeled
- 3 tablespoons of tahini
- zest of ½ lemon
- Ground sea salt, to taste
- juice of 1 lemon

Directions

- Preheat oven to 400°F.
- Bake the sweet potatoes on the middle oven rack for more than 45 minutes.
- Toss all of the other ingredients into a food processor as the potatoes are cooling.
- Add the sweet potatoes to the food processor once the skin is peeled.

- Blend well.
- Serve and enjoy with a light sprinkle of cayenne pepper and sesame seeds.

Vegetarian black bean and sweet potato enchilada

The potatoes are smothered in a salsa Verde with a delicious vegetarian entrée. It features various vegetables for a better taste and flavor.

Ingredients

- 4 ounces of grated cheese
- 1 ¼ pounds sweet potatoes
- 1 can of black beans, rinsed and drained
- 2 tablespoons sour cream
- ¼ cup chopped red onion
- 2 ounces of crumbled feta cheese
- 2 small cans of diced green chilies
- 1 medium jalapeño, seeded and minced
- 2 cloves garlic, pressed or minced
- 1 tablespoon water
- 2 tablespoons lime juice
- ¼ cup chopped fresh cilantro
- ½ teaspoon ground cumin
- ½ teaspoon chili powder
- ¼ teaspoon cayenne pepper

- ¼ teaspoon salt, more to taste
- Freshly ground black pepper
- 2 cups of mild salsa Verde
- 10 corn tortillas

Directions

- Preheat your oven ready to 400°F.
- Line a large baking sheet with parchment paper.
- Place the coated sweet potatoes with oil, flat-side down on the baking sheet.
- Bake for 35 minutes or until tender and cooked through.
- Pour enough salsa Verde into a baking dish to lightly cover the bottom
- In a medium mixing bowl, combine cumin, lime juice, cayenne pepper, chili powder, garlic, jalapeno, green chilies, feta cheese, jack cheese, beans, salt, and ground black pepper.
- Scoop out the potato flesh with a spoon. Lightly mash them with a fork.
- Stir the mashed sweet potato into the bowl of filling, and season to taste.

- Warm up your tortillas, in a skillet, wrap them in a clean tea towel to maintain the warmth.
- Working with one tortilla at a time, spread about ½ cup filling down the center each tortilla, then wrap both sides over the filling and place it in the baking dish.
- Repeat for all of the tortillas.
- Top with the remaining salsa Verde and cheese.
- Bake for 35 minutes, until sauce is bubbling.
- Let cool and drizzle with sour cream.
- Serve and enjoy.

Roasted vegetable enchilada casserole

Unlike other Mediterranean Sea diet recipes, this one takes a different turn of featuring hearty fresh Mexican vegetable flavors. It a main dish and gluten free.

Ingredients

- ½ cup of chopped fresh cilantro
- 10 corn tortillas, halved
- ½ medium head of cauliflower, cut into chunks
- 1 large sweet potato, peeled and cut into cubes
- Freshly ground black pepper
- 1 can of black beans, rinsed and drained
- 2 red bell peppers, cut into 1" squares
- 2 cups shredded Jack cheese
- 1 medium yellow onion, sliced into wedges
- 3 tablespoons of extra-virgin olive oil, divided
- 2 big handfuls of baby spinach leaves
- 1 teaspoon of ground cumin, divided
- Salt
- 2 ¼ cups of red salsa

Directions

- Preheat your oven ready to 400°F.
- Line 2 large, baking sheets with parchment paper.
- Combine the cauliflower and sweet potato in one pan.
- On the other, combine the bell peppers together with the onion.
- Drizzle half of the olive oil over one pan, and the other half over the other pan.
- Sprinkle them lightly with salt and pepper, toss to coat vegetables in oil and spices.
- Arrange the vegetables in an even layer across each pan.
- Let bake until the vegetables are tender on the edges, for 35 minutes, tossing and swapping the pans halfway.
- Lower the oven heat and lightly grease square baker. Then, stir the cilantro into the salsa.
- Spread ½ cup salsa evenly over the bottom of the baking pan.
- Add a single layer of halved tortilla pieces.

- Top with beans, vegetables, spinach, and ⅓ of the cheese.
- Make a second layer of tortillas topping with remaining components.
- Make many layers as you can.
- Cover the pan with parchment paper, let bake for 20 minutes, then remove the parchment paper, let bake for 10 more minutes.
- Serve and enjoy.

Mason jar chickpea, faro, and greens salad

Ingredients

- Handful of dried cherries
- 1 ¼ cup of faro
- ¼ cup of pepitas
- 1 tablespoon of olive oil
- 1 medium clove garlic, pressed or minced
- Kalamata olives, pitted and thinly sliced
- ¼ teaspoon salt
- ½ cup of red wine vinegar
- 4 cloves garlic, pressed or minced
- 4 stalks celery, thinly sliced and roughly chopped
- Feta cheese, crumbled
- 1 tablespoon of dried oregano
- 2 teaspoons of Dijon mustard
- ⅓ cup of Greek dressing
- 1 teaspoon of freshly ground black pepper
- 1 teaspoon of agave nectar, honey or sugar
- 2 cans of chickpeas, drained and rinsed

- ⅔ cup of chopped red onion
- 1 cup of chopped parsley
- Mixed greens

Directions

- In a medium saucepan, combine the rinsed faro together with 3 cups water
- Bring the water to a boil, then reduce heat to a gentle simmer, until the faro is tender.
- Drain any excess water and mix in the olive oil together with the garlic and salt. Let cool.
- Then, whisk together extra virgin olive oil, red wine vinegar, garlic, dried oregano, Dijon mustard, salt, ground black pepper, and agave nectar until emulsified.
- In a serving bowl, toss together the chickpeas together with the prepared celery, red onion, and parsley. Stir in enough dressing to coat the salad. Toss and set aside.
- In another skillet over medium heat, toast the pepitas for a few minutes, stirring frequently, until they smell toasty.
- Let cool in a bowl.

- In a quart-sized mason jar, layer the chickpea salad at the bottom with an additional tablespoon of dressing.
- Top with cooled faro and greens.
- Serve and enjoy.

Feta fiesta kale salad with avocado and crispy tortilla strips

This recipe combines broad ingredients ranging from vegetables and fruit juice with herbs. Therefore, it is a perfect choice of Mediterranean Sea diet.

Ingredients

- In a small bowl, whisk olive oil together with lime juice, jalapeno, honey, ground honey, coriander, and pinch of salt until emulsified.
- Place chopped and sliced kale to a big salad bowl.
- Sprinkle with a small pinch of sea salt, then massage the leaves with hands at a time, until the leaves turn darker and fragrant.
- Drizzle salad dressing over the kale and toss well t coat.
- Add the drained black beans together with the feta, avocado and chopped cilantro to mixing bowl.
- In a skillet over medium-low heat toast the pepitas for briefly, stirring frequently, until fragrant.

- Transfer to the salad bowl. Toss to combine.
- Stack the corn tortillas and slice them into thin little strips.
- Heat a large pan drizzled with olive oil over medium heat.
- Toss in the tortilla slices when the olive oil begins to shimmer, sprinkle with salt and stir.
- Let cook until the strips are crispy and turning golden in 5 minutes, stirring occasionally.
- Remove tortilla strips from skillet and drain on a plate covered with a piece of paper towel.
- Serve and enjoy topped with salad and crispy tortilla strips.

Thai mango cabbage wraps with crispy tofu and peanut sauce

The Thai mango cabbage wrap is a wonderfully delicious Mediterranean Sea diet recipe with healthy peanut sauce, cabbage as a salad wrap is irresistible.

Ingredients

- ⅓ cup of packed fresh cilantro leaves, chopped
- 1 block of organic extra-firm tofu
- 1 medium red bell pepper, chopped
- 1 jalapeño, minced
- 1 tablespoon of olive oil
- 2 garlic cloves, pressed
- ¼ teaspoon salt
- 1 tablespoon of reduced-sodium tamari
- 2 teaspoons of arrowroot
- 2 tablespoons large, [unsweetened coconut flakes]
- ⅓ cup of creamy peanut butter
- 2 tablespoons of white wine vinegar
- 2 tablespoons chopped peanuts
- 1 small head of green cabbage

- 2 tablespoons of honey
- 2 teaspoons of toasted sesame oil
- 1 lime, juiced
- 2 ripe mangos, diced
- ½ bunch of green onions, chopped

Directions

- Preheat your oven ready to 400°F.
- Drain the tofu completely.
- Slice tofu into thirds.
- Transfer to a plate lined with paper towels.
- Fold the towel over one tofu slab, then place the other slab on top.
- Repeat with the last slab.
- Whisk together peanut butter, white wine vinegar, tamari, honey, sesame oil, and garlic until well blended.
- Transfer the drained tofu to a cutting board.
- Slice each slab into four columns and four rows.
- Whisk together 1 tablespoon olive oil and tamari, then drizzle it over the tofu and toss to coat.

- Sprinkle 1 teaspoon arrowroot starch over the tofu, toss to incorporated.
- Let bake for 35 minutes, tossing, until the tofu is deeply golden.
- Combine mangos, red bell pepper, green onions, cilantro leaves, jalapeno, lime juice, and salt in a small serving bowl, toss.
- Pull off one leaf at a time. Repeat until you have 8 cabbage leaves.
- Toast the coconut flakes and chopped peanuts over medium heat, stirring frequently, until the coconut is golden.
- Add the tofu to the pan. Pour in the peanut sauce, toss to coat. Cook, until the tofu has absorbed the sauce.
- Serve and enjoy.

Strawberry kale salad with nutty granola croutons

A combination of raw vegetables and fruits mainly red kale, strawberries, radishes with crumbled cheese is healthy for any individual.

Ingredients

- ½ cup of raw sunflower seeds
- 8 ounces of kale
- ½ cup of whole almonds
- ¼ cup of raw sesame seeds
- ½ pound of strawberries, hulled and sliced
- 5 medium radishes, sliced thin and roughly chopped
- 1 tablespoon of fennel seeds
- 2 ounces of chilled goat cheese
- 1 cup of old-fashioned oats
- ¼ teaspoon of cayenne pepper
- 3 tablespoons of olive oil
- 2 tablespoons of lemon juice
- 1 tablespoon of smooth Dijon mustard
- 1 large egg white, beaten

- 2 ½ teaspoons of honey
- Sea salt and freshly ground pepper, to taste
- ½ cup of raw shelled pistachios

Directions

- Preheat oven to 350°F.
- Then, in a medium bowl, toss oats together with the sunflower seeds, sesame seeds, fennel seeds, pistachios, almonds, salt, and cayenne pepper.
- Stir in the beaten egg white with olive oil, and honey, until blended.
- Transfer mixture to baking sheet.
- Let bake, stirring halfway, until golden in 19 minutes. Allow it to cool on the baking sheet.
- In another small mixing bowl, whisk together the olive oil with lemon juice, mustard, and honey until emulsified.
- Season with sea salt and freshly ground black pepper.
- Transfer the chopped kale to a big salad bowl.
- Sprinkle with a small pinch of sea salt and massage the leaves with your hands.

- Drizzle in the salad dressing, toss well, until all of the kale is lightly coated in dressing.
- Add the sliced strawberries and chopped radishes, then use a fork to crumble the goat cheese over the salad.
- Serve and enjoy.

Sugar snap pea and carrot soba noodles

The sugar snap pea and carrot soba noodles recipe features a highly vibrant fresh springtime produce good enough for a Mediterranean Sea diet.

Ingredients

- 1 tablespoon of white miso
- 6 ounces of [soba noodles](#)
- 2 cups of frozen organic edamame
- 10 ounces of sugar snap peas
- 1 tablespoon of toasted sesame oil
- 6 medium-sized carrots, peeled
- 1 tablespoon of honey
- 1 teaspoon of chili garlic sauce
- ½ cup of chopped fresh cilantro
- 1 small lime, juiced
- ¼ cup of sesame seeds
- 2 teaspoons of freshly grated ginger
- ¼ cup of reduced-sodium tamari
- 2 tablespoons of peanut oil

Directions

- Whisk together tamari, peanut oil, lemon juice, sesame oil, honey, white miso, ginger, and chili garlic sauce in a small bowl until emulsified. Keep aside for later.
- Bring 2 big pots of water to a boil.
- As the water boils, pour the sesame seeds into a small pan. Toast for 5 minutes over medium heat, shaking the pan frequently, until the seeds are turning golden.
- Cook the soba noodles according to package Directions in the boiling water.
- Drain any excess water and rinse under cool water.
- Then, cook the frozen edamame in the other pot until warmed through in 6 minutes.
- Toss the halved peas into the boiling edamame water and cook for an additional 20 seconds. Drain.
- Combine the soba noodles together with the edamame, snap peas, and carrots in a large serving bowl.

- Pour in the dressing, toss with salad servers.
- Serve and enjoy tossed in the chopped cilantro and toasted sesame seeds. Serve.

Lemony lentil and chickpea salad with radish and herbs

This recipe blends beans with lemon and mint flavor. It takes only 20 minutes for the chickpea and lentils to get ready for your lunch or dinner.

Ingredients

- 2 cups of dried black beluga lentils
- 1 big bunch of radishes, sliced thin and roughly chopped
- Freshly ground black pepper, to taste
- 2 large garlic cloves, halved lengthwise
- ¼ cup of chopped fresh, leafy herbs, chopped
- 1 clove of garlic, pressed or minced
- 4 tablespoons of olive oil
- 1 can of chickpeas, rinsed and drained
- ¼ cup of fresh lemon juice
- Sliced avocado, crumbled feta
- 1 teaspoon of Dijon mustard
- 1 teaspoon of honey
- ¼ teaspoon of fine-grain sea salt

Directions

- In a medium pot, combine the lentils together with garlic cloves, olive oil and 4 cups water.
- Bring the water to a boil, then lower the heat, let simmer and cook until the lentils tender in 35 minutes max.
- Drain the lentils and discard the garlic cloves.
- Whisk together the chickpeas, radishes, fresh herbs, and avocado slices in a small bowl.
- In a large serving bowl, combine the lentils together with the chickpeas, chopped radishes and herbs.
- Drizzle in the dressing and toss to combine.
- Serve and enjoy with avocado, crumbled cheese and or fresh greens.

Roasted cherry tomato, arugula and sorghum salad

The presence of sorghum makes this recipe quite unique and truly Mediterranean with other various vegetables with a lemon dressing. It is quite healthy; the sorghum is a greater source of carbohydrates as the chickpea is a greater source of proteins.

Ingredients

- 3 cups of baby arugula
- 1 cup of sorghum, rinsed
- ¼ cup of crumbled feta
- 3 cups of water
- 1 can of chickpeas, rinsed and drained
- ¼ teaspoon of fine grain sea salt
- 1 pint of cherry tomatoes
- Sea salt
- 3 tablespoons olive oil
- 2 tablespoons of lemon juice
- 2 tablespoons of grated Parmesan cheese
- ¼ teaspoon of red pepper flakes
- 1 clove of garlic, pressed

- Freshly ground black pepper, to taste

Directions

- Combine rinsed sorghum with water in a small pot.
- Bring to a boil, covered, then lower the heat to medium-low.
- Cook until the sorghum is pleasantly tender In 66 minutes.
- Then, preheat your oven to 400°F.
- Line a small, baking sheet with parchment paper.
- Toss the whole cherry tomatoes with 1 tablespoon of olive oil, then sprinkle with salt.
- Let, roast for 18 minutes, or until the tomatoes are plump and starting to burst open.
- Whisk together the red pepper flakes, olive oil, lemon juice, salt and pepper until emulsified.
- Drain off any excess water out of the sorghum, pour into a serving bowl.
- Pour in all of the dressing, all of the cherry tomatoes and their juices, the arugula, feta,

Parmesan and chickpeas, then, give it a big toss.

- Serve and enjoy.

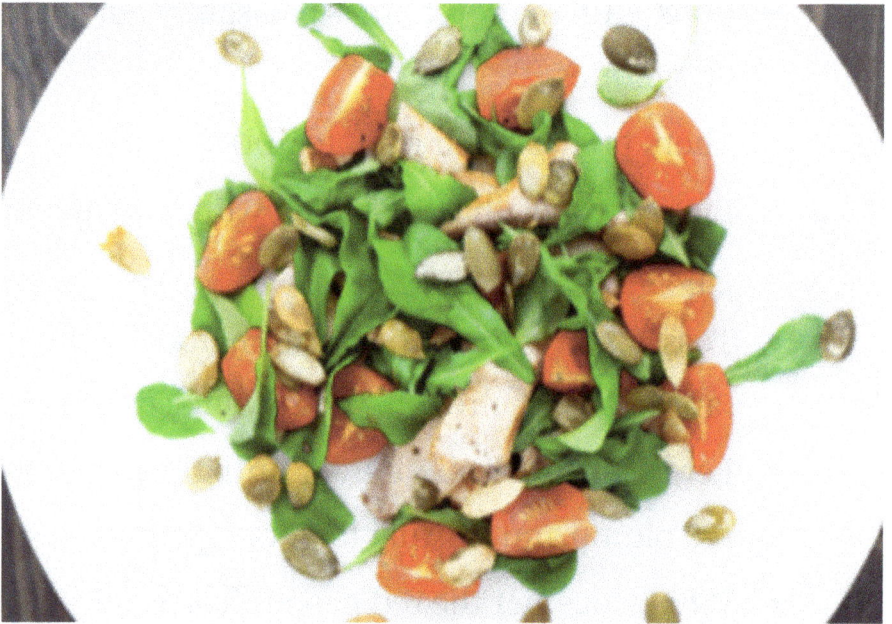

Spring carrot, radish, and quinoa salad with herbed avocado

In a simple lemon vinaigrette, this recipe features several vegetables such as carrots, fennel, garlicky, radishes, quinoa, and herbed avocado for a perfect Mediterranean Sea diet choice.

Ingredients

- 2 garlic cloves, pressed or minced
- 1 small lime or lemon, juiced
- 2 ½ teaspoons of olive oil
- 3 packed tablespoons of fresh herbs
- 4 cups of arugula
- ⅛ teaspoon of sea salt
- 2 radishes, sliced into strips
- Lots of freshly ground black pepper
- 3 carrots, peeled and then sliced into ribbons
- ¼ bulb fennel, cored and sliced thinly
- 3 tablespoons of sunflower seeds
- 3 tablespoons of crumbled feta
- 1 lemon, zested and juiced
- Dash sea salt

- ½ cup of quinoa, rinsed
- ½ teaspoon o ground coriander
- 1 teaspoon of Dijon mustard
- ½ teaspoon honey or agave nectar
- 1 large avocado, diced

Directions

- In a saucepan, combine the quinoa and 1 cup water.
- Bring the mixture to a boil, covered, then lower the heat to a simmer.
- Let cook for 15 minutes, remove let it rest, for 5 minutes.
- Fluff the quinoa and mix in the garlic with the olive oil.
- Season, and adjust accordingly.
- Pour the seeds into a small pan.
- Heat the seeds over medium heat, stirring frequently, until turning golden on the edges. Remove.
- In a small bowl, whisk the olive oil together with the lemon juice and zest, mustard, and honey until emulsified.

- Season with sea salt and black pepper.
- In another separate small bowl, combine the chunks of avocado, chopped fresh herbs, lemon or lime juice, coriander, and sea salt.
- Mash with a fork until the mixture is blended.
- Divide the arugula and quinoa between two large salad bowls.
- Then, drizzle with vinaigrette lightly, and toss to coat.
- Divide the radishes, carrots, and fennel between the two bowls.
- Top with a sprinkling of sunflower seeds and feta cheese.
- Serve and enjoy.

Kale, clementine, and feta salad with honey lime dressing

Everything else is toasted in natural honey; the raw kale salad, radish, avocado, clementine, and peppitas making it a perfect choice for a vegetarian Mediterranean Sea diet choice.

Ingredients

- ¼ teaspoon of chili powder
- 1 bunch of kale
- 1 teaspoon of Dijon mustard
- 1 avocado, diced
- 3 tablespoons of olive oil
- 1 medium pomegranate, arils removed
- ⅛ teaspoon of fine grain sea salt
- 2 teaspoons of honey
- 4 clementine, peeled and sliced into rounds
- 1 medium jalapeño
- 4 small radishes, sliced into thin rounds
- Handful of fresh cilantro, chopped
- ⅓ cup of crumbled feta
- ¼ cup of pepitas

- 3 tablespoons of fresh lime juice

Directions

- Firstly, whisk fresh lime juice together with olive oil, jalapeno, honey, Dijon mustard, chili powder, and grain sea salt in a small bowl.
- Place sliced kale into a big salad bowl.
- Sprinkle a small pinch of sea salt and massage the leaves with your hands by lightly scrunching.
- Drizzle salad dressing over the kale, toss well to coat with dressing.
- Add the prepared avocado, clementine, radishes, pomegranate, cilantro, and feta to the bowl.
- In a skillet over medium-low heat toast the pepitas briefly, stirring frequently, until fragrant.
- Transfer the pepitas to the salad bowl. Toss to combine.
- Serve and enjoy.

Lemon parsley bean salad

This deliciously irresistible recipe draws its flavor and aroma from the garlic, red onion, and herbs. It is totally vegan with plenty of vegetables, herbs, and lemon juice.

Ingredients

- ¾ teaspoon of salt
- 2 cans of red kidney beans, rinsed and drained
- 1 can of chickpeas, rinsed and drained
- 3 cloves garlic, pressed
- 1 small red onion, diced
- ¼ cup of lemon juice
- Small pinch of red pepper flakes
- 2 stalks celery, sliced in half
- 1 medium cucumber, peeled, seeded and diced
- ¾ cup of chopped fresh parsley
- 2 tablespoons of chopped fresh dill
- ¼ cup of olive oil

Directions

- In a serving bowl, combine the prepared kidney beans together with the chickpeas, onion, celery, cucumber, parsley, and dill.

- In another separate small bowl, whisk together the olive oil, lemon juice, garlic, salt and pepper flakes until emulsified.
- Pour dressing over the bean and vegetable mixture, toss well.
- Place to marinate in the refrigerator for hours.
- Or serve and enjoy immediately.

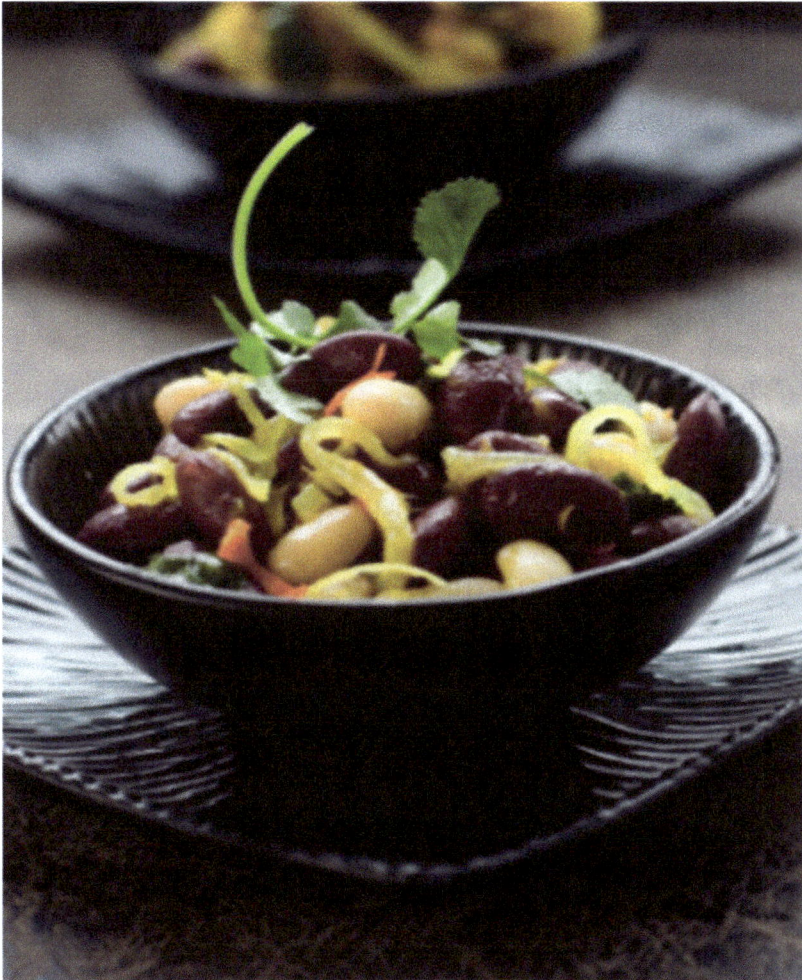

Lemon parsley hummus with baked pita chips

This recipe can be used as a snack for an appetizer packed with herbs and vegetables for a wonderful and delicious Mediterranean Sea diet.

Ingredients

- Olive oil
- 1½ cans of chickpeas, rinsed and drained
- Dash freshly ground black pepper
- Fine grain sea salt
- ⅓ cup of fresh lemon juice
- ¾ cup of chopped parsley
- ¼ cup of tahini
- Whole grain pita bread
- 5 cloves of garlic, roughly chopped
- ¼ teaspoon of fine grain sea salt
- 1 tablespoon of olive oil

Directions

- In a food processor, combine the chickpeas together with the tahini, garlic, lemon juice, parsley, sea salt and black pepper.

- Turn on the food processor, then drizzle in 1 tablespoon olive oil.
- Process until the hummus is creamy and relatively smooth.
- Add salt to taste.
- Transfer to a serving bowl and top with a light drizzle of olive oil.
- Preheat your oven ready to 400°F.
- Slice the pita bread into small wedges.
- Brush with olive oil on both sides.
- Sprinkle with sea salt.
- Then, let bake for 10 minutes, flipping halfway, or until crisp and lightly golden.
- Serve and enjoy.

Summer squash salad with lemon citronette

Ingredients

- 1 teaspoon of chopped fresh mint
- ¼ cup of pine nuts
- 1 teaspoon of chopped fresh flat-leaf parsley
- 1 tablespoon of fresh lemon juice
- 2 pounds of mixed baby zucchini and yellow squash
- Salt
- 1 cup of feta cheese, crumbled
- 1 teaspoon of chopped fresh thyme
- 3 tablespoons of olive oil
- ½ teaspoon of finely grated lemon zest
- 1 large garlic clove, pressed or minced

Directions

- Spread squash ribbons on a cutting board.
- Sprinkle with salt, and let them sit for 20 minutes.

- In a small skillet over medium-low heat, toast the nuts until turning golden and fragrant, stirring frequently.
- In another separate small bowl, whisk together the lemon zest and juice with garlic, thyme, mint, and parsley.
- As it is whisking, drizzle in the olive oil until the dressing is well blended. Set aside for later.
- Rinse and pat dry the squash.
- Place in a serving bowl, then before serving, whisk the citronette last time.
- Toss the squash with the feta, pine nuts and citronette.
- Serve and enjoy immediately.

The little green salad

Ingredients

- Sliced cherry tomatoes, avocado and sunflower seeds
- Arugula
- Freshly ground black pepper, to taste
- Small nuts, toasted
- Freshly grated Parmesan
- Thinly sliced fennel and pine nuts
- ¼ cup of olive oil
- 2 tablespoons of lemon juice
- Thinly sliced cucumbers, radishes and almonds
- 2 teaspoons of Dijon mustard
- Pinch of sea salt

Directions

- Start by whisking together the olive oil, lemon juice, Dijon mustard, sea salt and ground black pepper in a small bowl until well blended.

- In another mixing bowl, combine the arugula with a handful of toasted nuts and grated Parmesan.
- Add a drizzle of dressing and toss until the salad is lightly coated throughout.
- Serve and enjoy after tossing.

Spicy sun dried tomato and broccoli pasta

Ingredients

- Bring a large pot of salted water to a boil.
- Add the pasta to the boiling water, cook as directed on the package Directions.
- Drain any excess water, reserving some for later.
- In a large non-stick skillet, heat 3 tablespoons of olive oil over medium heat.
- Add the red pepper flakes and garlic, cook, stirring constantly, until the garlic begins to simmer.
- Pour and scrape the seasoned oil into the heatproof bowl and set aside.
- Add 2 tablespoons of olive oil, heat over medium temperature until shimmering.
- Then, add the broccoli sprinkled with 1 teaspoon salt.
- Cook, stirring occasionally, until the broccoli has shrunk to a single layer.
- Add the sun-dried tomatoes to the pan. Pour ⅓ cup pasta water into the pan. Cover and

continue cooking until the water has simmered down to almost nothing in 40 seconds.

- Add the drained pasta to the pan and drizzle in all of the infused oil.
- Stir in the goat cheese with Parmigiano.
- Add another 2 tablespoons of pasta water with chopped olives and lemon juice, and stir until the goat cheese loosens up.
- Season with salt accordingly.
- Serve and enjoy garnished with the remaining Parmigiano.

Blackened green bean and quinoa salad

Ingredients

- Sea salt and black pepper
- 1 cup of quinoa
- 2 teaspoons of Dijon mustard
- 2 corn on the cobs, stripped
- ⅓ cup sliced almonds
- 1 pound long green beans
- Salt and pepper
- 3 garlic cloves, mince
- ¼ cup of water
- Crumbled feta
- ½ medium red onion, sliced into thin strips
- 1 cup of cherry tomatoes, chopped
- ¼ cup of olive oil
- 2 small lemons, juiced
- 1 tablespoon of chopped fresh basil

Directions

- In a medium saucepan, combine 2 cups water with quinoa.

- Bring to a boil, let simmer for 17 minutes, covered until the water is absorbed.
- Remove from heat, fluff with a fork, set aside.
- Then, heat 2 teaspoons of olive oil in over medium heat until shimmering.
- Add the green beans sprinkled with salt, cook, for 6 minutes, stirring occasionally, until spotty brown.
- Add another teaspoon olive oil with minced garlic.
- Let cook until fragrant, then, Stir the garlic into the green beans.
- Add the red onion the pan, with water and cover until the beans are bright green and crisp.
- Uncover, raise the heat to medium-high.
- Cook until the water evaporates and the beans are lightly browned.
- Transfer to a big mixing bowl.
- Add the cooked quinoa, chopped cherry tomatoes, and corn kernels.

- Whisk together the dressing ingredients in a small bowl and pour it into the salad bowl. Toss to combine.
- Season with salt and flaky pepper.
- In a skillet over medium-low heat, toast the almond slivers until fragrant and golden.
- Serve and enjoy with toasted almonds and feta.

Kale salad with apple, cranberries, and pecans

Ingredients

- 1 tablespoon of smooth Dijon mustard
- ½ cup of pecans
- 1 ½ teaspoons of honey
- 1 ½ tablespoons of apple cider vinegar
- 3 tablespoons of olive oil
- 8 ounces of kale
- 5 medium radishes
- Sea salt and freshly ground pepper
- ½ cup of dried cranberries
- 1 medium Granny Smith apple
- 2 ounces of soft goat cheese, chilled

Directions

- Preheat your oven ready to 350°F.
- Then, spread the pecans on a baking tray. Toast lightly golden and fragrant in 10 minutes or so.
- Remove the tray, let to cool.
- Transfer the chopped kale to a big salad bowl.

- Sprinkle with a small pinch of sea salt, then massage the leaves with your hands.
- Add sliced radishes to the bowl.
- Add coarsely chop pecans, cranberries, and apples to the bowl. Crumble the goat cheese over the top.
- In a small bowl, whisk olive oil together with the apple cider vinegar, Dijon mustard, honey, sea salt and pepper, and pour over the salad.
- Toss to coat with dressing.
- Serve and enjoy immediately.

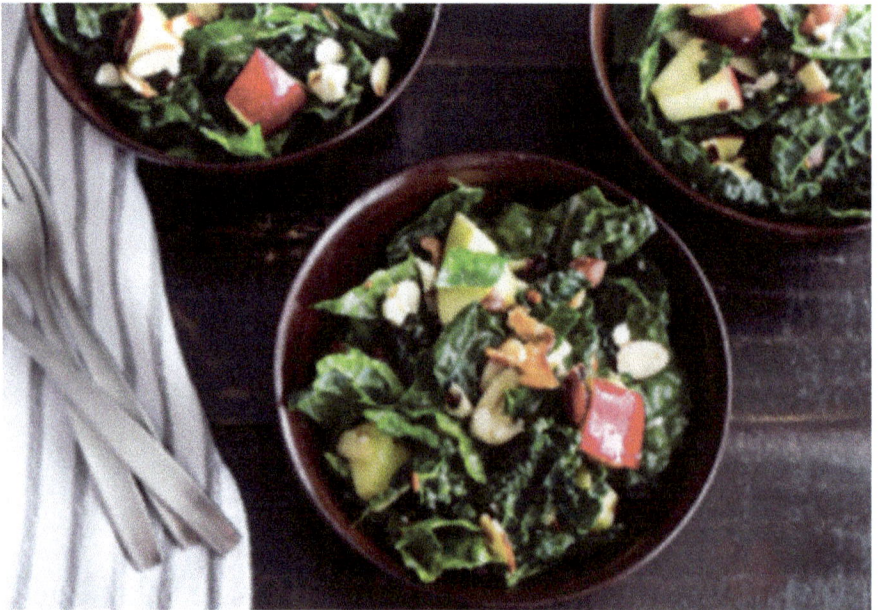

Orange, apricot, and carrot couscous

The orange, apricot, and carrot couscous recipe blends crunchy and tangy winter flavors for a better Mediterranean dish taste.

Ingredients

- ¼ medium-sized red onion
- 1 cup of whole-wheat couscous
- 1 medium carrot
- 2 teaspoons of grated fresh ginger
- ½ cup of water
- 1 cup of orange juice
- 2 tablespoons of dried currants or raisins
- ¼ cup of pine nuts
- 10 dried apricots, thinly sliced
- ¼ cup of extra-virgin olive oil
- 5 teaspoons of plum vinegar
- Sea salt

Directions

- Pour couscous into a medium-sized bowl, set aside.

- In a small pot, combine water together with the olive oil, orange juice, 4 teaspoons vinegar, and a pinch of sea salt.
- Bring the mixture to a boil, then add the dried fruit and ginger. Let simmer for briefly.
- Stir, then pour the liquid mixture over the dry couscous.
- Stir to remove any pockets of dry couscous.
- Peel the carrot into ribbons over the couscous, then cover the concoction with a plate to trap the heat.
- Toss onions with 1 teaspoon vinegar in a small bowl.
- In another separate small pan, toast the pine nuts until lightly golden over medium heat, tossing frequently.
- Serve and enjoy chilled or warm.

Sumer rolls with spicy peanut sauce

Ingredients

- ⅓ cup chopped fresh cilantro
- ½ cup of roasted peanuts
- ⅓ cup chopped fresh mint
- ½ cup of light coconut milk
- 8 sheets rice paper
- 2 red bell peppers
- 2 tablespoons of lime juice
- 1 tablespoon of agave nectar
- Sriracha hot sauce
- 1 tablespoon of reduced sodium tamari
- 5 cloves garlic
- Pinch of red pepper flakes
- 3 green onions, sliced into thin rounds
- 1 package of extra-firm tofu
- 2 tablespoon of sesame seeds
- 2 heaping cups of arugula, roughly chopped
- 3 big carrots
- 4 Persian cucumbers
- 1 jalapeño, cut into matchsticks

Directions

- In a food processor, process roasted peanuts, coconut milk, lime juice, agave nectar, tamari, garlic, and red pepper, until fairly smooth.
- Transfer to a small bowl.
- Stack tofu slabs on top of each other and place a heavy saucepan on top.
- Slice each tofu slab into 7 equal-sized strips.
- Sprinkle with sesame seeds onto a plate, roll the tofu strips to coat.
- Fill a baking pan with warm water.
- Place one rice paper in the water and let it rest for about twenty seconds. Lay it on the towel.
- Top the rice paper with a big sprinkle of arugula, a few strips of carrot, one strip of tofu, cucumber, bell pepper, and jalapeño.
- Sprinkle with some chopped green onion, cilantro and mint.
- Fold over one long side to enclose the filling, then fold over the short sides and lastly, roll it up.
- Serve and enjoy.

Coconut quinoa and kale with tropical pesto

Ingredients

- Salt and freshly ground black pepper, to taste
- 1 cup of quinoa, rinsed
- ½ cup of olive oil
- 1 cup of light coconut milk
- ½ lime, juiced
- 4 cloves garlic
- 1 small bunch of kale
- ⅓ cup of chopped red onion
- pinch red pepper flakes
- ⅓ cup of large, unsweetened coconut flakes
- 2 cups of cilantro, packed
- Scant ½ cup of raw, unsalted cashews

Directions

- Combine coconut milk with water in a medium sized saucepan, bring to a boil.
- Add the quinoa, and simmer covered for 17 minutes, until the water is absorbed.

- Remove, fluff with a fork and mix in the red onion. Set aside.
- Combine cilantro together with the cashews and garlic in a food processor.
- Processing the mixture as you slowly drizzle in the olive oil.
- Season with salt, pepper, lime juice and red pepper flakes, and blend well.
- In a medium serving bowl, combine the warm coconut quinoa, chopped kale and pesto.
- Mix well with a big spoon.
- Taste, and adjust the seasoning
- In a skillet over medium heat, toast the coconut flakes briefly until golden, stirring often.
- Serve and enjoy topped with coconut flakes.

Stacked tomato, summer vegetable, and grilled bread salad

The stacked tomato, summer vegetable recipe is a great Mediterranean Sea diet with an array of vegetables and herbs which are beautifully grilled.

Ingredients

- Thick slices of whole wheat peasant bread
- 1 cup of sliced cherry tomatoes
- 4 tablespoons of olive oil
- 2 tablespoons of finely chopped and drained oil-packed sun-dried tomatoes
- Sea salt
- 1 tablespoon of red wine vinegar
- 3 cups of baby arugula leaves
- 1 tablespoon of lemon juice
- 1 tablespoon of chopped fresh mint and basil
- 4 ounces of goat cheese
- 2 large zucchini
- 1 teaspoon of honey
- ½ teaspoon of finely chopped Kalamata olives
- 2 red bell peppers

- ½ teaspoon of minced fresh garlic
- ¼ teaspoon of ground sea salt

Directions

- In a small bowl, whisk olive oil, sundried tomatoes, red wine vinegar, lemon juice, mint and basil, honey, Kalamata olives, garlic, and sea salt.
- Fold in the tomatoes, let rest.
- Hold red bell peppers directly over the flame of a gas stove, until the peppers are blackened.
- Transfer the peppers to a bowl and cover tightly, let cool for 20 minutes, and peel, and cut.
- Reduce the grill heat to medium.
- Brush zucchini slices on both sides with olive oil and sprinkle with salt.
- Brush slices of bread with olive oil on both sides and sprinkle with salt.
- Arrange the bread slices and zucchini pieces in a single layer on the grill and close the lid.
- Let until golden brown on both sides. Meanwhile cook the zucchini until well-

marked on the first side for 5 minutes, then flip and cook the same way.

- Transfer the zucchini to a plate and cover loosely to retain heat.
- Rub the grilled bread on both sides with the garlic clove.
- Serve and enjoy sprinkled with herbs and scattered lettuce leaves.

Sweet corn salad wraps

Ingredients

- 6 ears of fresh corn, kernels removed
- 1 small red onion, chopped finely
- ½ red bell pepper, chopped
- Handful of cherry tomatoes
- ½ cup of chopped fresh cilantro
- 1 teaspoon of ancho chili powder
- pinch of cayenne pepper
- 2 small limes, juiced
- Sea salt and black pepper
- 1 teaspoon of olive oil
- 1 head of white cabbage
- 2 small corn tortillas
- 1 avocado

Directions

- Start by combining the raw corn kernels together with the onion, cherry tomatoes, cilantro, bell pepper, chili powder, cayenne pepper, and the juice of limes in a mixing bowl.
- Season with salt and pepper.

- Place each leaf of cabbage on its own in a small plate.
- In a small skillet, on medium-high heat, pour in enough oil to form a thin film on the surface.
- Then, add the tortilla strips, sprinkled with bit of salt, let fry until crisp, stirring occasionally.
- Remove tortilla strips from skillet and drain.
- Spoon about ½ cup of the salsa mixture onto each leaf, then top with crispy tortilla strips and avocado.
- Serve and enjoy immediately.

Raw kale salad with creamy tahini dressing

Ingredients

- Dash of tamari or soy sauce
- 1 bunch of curly kale
- Sea salt
- Big pinch red pepper flakes
- ⅓ cup of water
- 1 avocado
- 6 carrots
- Small handful of chopped cilantro
- 2 teaspoons of sesame seeds
- ¼ cup tahini
- 1 tablespoon of white miso
- 1 ½ tablespoons of rice vinegar
- ½ teaspoon toasted sesame oil

Directions

- Sprinkle a small pinch of sea salt over the prepared kale and massage the leaves briefly.

- In a small bowl, whisk together the tahini, white miso, rice vinegar, sesame oil, red pepper flakes, water, and tamari.
- Divide the kale into two bowls, drizzle in the salad dressing, toss thoroughly.
- Top the salad with carrot ribbons, diced avocado, and some chopped carrot greens.
- Serve and enjoy.

Saladu nebbe

Ingredients

- 2 serrano peppers or 1 habanero
- ¼ cup of fresh lime juice
- 1 cup of chopped parsley
- 1 medium cucumber, seeded and finely chopped
- Sliced avocado
- ½ cup of olive oil
- 5 cups of cooked black-eyed peas
- Cooked brown basmati rice
- 10 scallions, roughly chopped
- 1 red bell pepper, stemmed, seeded, and finely chopped
- 1 cup cherry, chopped
- Sea salt and freshly ground black pepper, to taste

Directions

- In a large bowl, whisk together the lime juice with the parsley.
- Keep whisking as you drizzle in the olive oil to make a smooth dressing.

- Add the black-eyed peas together with the scallions, bell pepper, tomato, cucumber, and minced pepper to the bowl.
- Season the mixture with salt and pepper, toss the salad.
- Pack well and refrigerate overnight for a better taste.
- Serve and enjoy on top of cooked brown basmati rice topped with avocado slices.

Wheat berries

Ingredients

- ½ teaspoon of ground sea salt
- 1 cup of dried wheat berries
- ¼ teaspoon of red pepper flakes
- 2 cups of cooked chickpeas
- 4 carrots
- 1 small lemon, juiced
- ⅓ cup of olive oil
- Ground black pepper, to taste
- ½ cup of feta cheese, crumbled
- 6 cups of arugula
- 2 teaspoons of honey
- 2 garlic cloves, pressed

Directions

- Bring 4 quarts of water to a boil in a large pot.
- Stir in the wheat berries with salt.
- Cover the pot halfway, let cook, stirring often, until the berries are tender.
- Drain the wheat berries, let cool to room temperature.

- Then, whisk olive oil together with the honey, garlic, red pepper flakes, lemon juice, sea salt, and black pepper.
- Transfer the cooled wheat berries to a big bowl.
- Add the chickpeas together with the carrots, feta cheese, and arugula, toss to combine.
- Drizzle in the dressing and toss to coat.
- Serve and enjoy warm.

Ribboned asparagus and quinoa salad

Ingredients

- 2 tablespoons of pine nuts
- 1 cup of cooked quinoa
- 7 stalks of asparagus
- 2 ounces of Parmesan, shaved
- Black pepper, to taste
- 1 small lemon
- olive oil
- Sea salt, to taste

Directions

- Combine rinsed quinoa with enough water in a saucepan.
- Bring to a boil, cover and reduce heat to a simmer.
- Let cook for 15 minutes to absorbed all the water.
- In a skillet over medium heat, stirring often, toast the pine nut for 10 minutes.
- In a bowl, combine cooked quinoa together with the shaved asparagus.
- Squeeze in most of the juice of half a lemon.

- Drizzle with olive oil.
- Sprinkle with sea salt and ground black pepper, toss to coat.
- Sprinkle with the pine nuts.
- Serve and enjoy.

Watercress and forbidden rice salad with ginger vinaigrette

Ingredients

- 3 stalks of celery, thinly sliced
- 1-inch nub of ginger, grated or finely chopped
- ¼ cup of green onion, chopped
- 3 cloves garlic, pressed
- 2 tablespoons of rice wine vinegar
- 1 ½ cups of cooked forbidden rice
- 1 yellow bell pepper, chopped
- ¼ cup of peanut oil, olive oil
- 2 teaspoons of toasted sesame oil
- 2 ½ teaspoons of reduced-sodium tamari
- 1 ½ cups of shelled edamame
- ½ teaspoon of agave nectar
- Pinch red pepper flakes
- 1 big bunch watercress

Directions

- Whisk ginger, garlic, rice wine vinegar, peanut oil, sesame oil, tamari, agave nectar, and red pepper flakes all together, set aside.

- Cook rice as instructed on the package.
- Bring a pot of water to a boil and pour in frozen edamame.
- Lower the heat to a simmer and cook until the edamame is warmed through in just 5 minutes.
- Drain, set aside to cool.
- Toss all of the prepared produce in a big bowl.
- Once the edamame and rice have cooled, add them to the bowl and toss.
- Serve and enjoy chilled.

Apple slaw for winter

This Mediterranean Sea diet apple recipe features a crunchy cabbage, tasty for any fruit or even vegetable lover for a breakfast.

Ingredients

- 2 medium apples
- Scant ¼ cup of olive oil
- ½ cup chopped cilantro
- 2 teaspoons of Dijon mustard
- 1 tablespoon of honey
- 1 lime, juiced
- Sea salt and pepper, to taste
- 1 small purple cabbage
- 8 radishes, stems and ends removed

Directions

- In a big bowl, whisk together olive oil with mustard, honey and lime juice.
- Toss the chopped cabbage, radish, and apple into the bowl.
- Toss the chopped ingredients with the dressing using a hand.

- Then, add salt and pepper, to taste.

- Cover and refrigerate for an hour.

- Mix in the chopped cilantro.

- Serve and enjoy immediately.

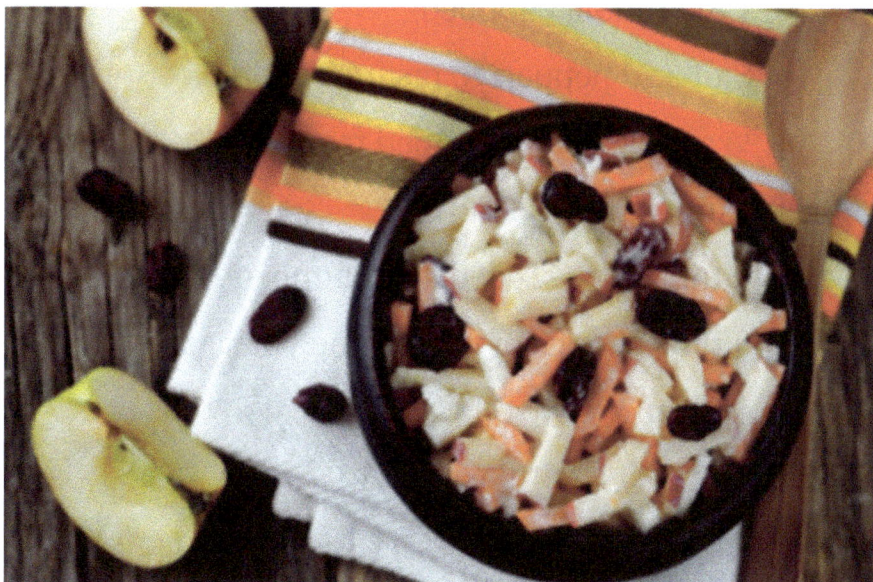

Cucumber dill salad

This a perfectly refreshing Mediterranean Sea diet recipe on its own as a standalone, yet incredibly tasty drawing its flavor from garlic, onions and herbs.

Ingredients

- ½ cup of crumbled feta cheese
- 1 teaspoon of minced garlic
- 3 cucumbers, seeded and chopped
- 1 red onion, chopped
- Salt and pepper, to taste
- ⅓ cup of finely chopped fresh dill
- 1 lime, juiced
- 3 tomatoes, seeded and chopped
- 3 tablespoons of white wine vinegar
- ¼ cup of olive oil

Directions

- In a large bowl, toss all of the ingredients together.
- Season with salt and pepper.
- Refrigerate for hours to circulate in the flavors.
- Serve and enjoy.

Vegan sour cream

If you are a vegan having challenges in identifying a recipe that suits your taste and preference, then look no further. Vegan sour cream is gluten free and it features herbs, vegetables and fruits.

Ingredients

- ¼ teaspoon of Dijon mustard
- ½ cup of water
- Heaping ¼ teaspoon of fine sea salt
- 1 cup of raw cashews
- 1 tablespoon of lemon juice
- 1 teaspoon of apple cider vinegar

Directions

- In a blender, combine the cashews together with water, lemon juice, vinegar, salt, and mustard.
- Blend until the mixture is smooth and creamy.
- Taste, and adjust the seasoning accordingly to your preference.
- Serve and enjoy immediately or chill the sour cream for later.

Arugula, apples, and Manchego in cider vinaigrette recipe

This is a Spanish Mediterranean diet style. It blends peppery arugula, juicy apples, Manchego with crunchy almonds then tossed in a cider vinaigrette.

Ingredients

- 1 teaspoon of Dijon mustard
- 1/4 teaspoon of ground black pepper
- 1 crisp apple
- 3 1/2 ounces of Manchego, thinly sliced
- 1/2 cup of sliced almonds
- 2 tablespoons of cider vinegar
- Heaping 1/4 teaspoon of salt
- 6 tablespoons of vegetable oil
- 5 ounces of arugula
- 2 teaspoons of maple syrup
- 1 tablespoon of chopped shallots

Directions

- Begin by whisking cider vinegar, vegetable oil, maple syrup, Dijon mustard, shallots, salt and ground black pepper in a small bowl. Set aside.

- Place arugula in serving bowl.
- Whisk the vinaigrette again until well combined, add the salad, little by little, until greens are well dressed.
- Slice the apple and toss into salad with Manchego and almonds.
- Taste and adjust seasoning.
- Serve and enjoy.

Healthy apple muffins

Ingredients

- ½ cup of plain Greek yogurt
- 1 ¾ cups of white whole wheat flour
- ½ cup of applesauce
- 1 ½ teaspoons of baking powder
- 1 teaspoon of vanilla extract
- 1 teaspoon of ground cinnamon
- ½ teaspoon of baking soda
- 1 tablespoon of turbinado sugar
- ½ teaspoon of salt
- 1 cup of grated apple
- 1 cup of apple diced into cubes
- ⅓ cup of melted coconut oil
- ½ cup of maple syrup
- 2 eggs

Directions

- Preheat your oven to 425°F.
- Grease 12 cups on the muffin tin with butter.

- In a large mixing bowl, combine the flour together with the baking powder, cinnamon, baking soda, and salt. Blend well.
- Add the grated apple with chopped apple. Stir to combine.
- In another separate medium mixing bowl, combine the oil together with maple syrup and whisk.
- Add the eggs and beat well.
- Add the yogurt, applesauce, and vanilla, mix well.
- Mix the wet ingredients with the dry ones, and mix to combined.
- Sprinkle the tops of the muffins with turbinado sugar.
- Let bake for 16 minutes, or until the muffins are golden on top.
- Place the muffin tin on a cooling rack to cool.
- Serve and enjoy.

Vibrant orange and arugula salad

Ingredients

- ¼ teaspoon of salt
- 3 tablespoons of lemon juice
- 6 ounces of baby arugula
- 2 oranges, peeled and sliced
- 1 ½ teaspoons of honey
- 2 ounces of goat cheese, crumbled
- Pinch of ground cinnamon
- ¼ cup of extra-virgin olive oil
- ¼ cup of thinly sliced radishes
- ¼ cup of sliced almonds

Directions

- In a small skillet warm the almonds over medium heat until fragrant in 5 minutes.
- Transfer to a bowl, let cool.
- Place the arugula on a large serving platter.
- Organize the oranges with toasted almonds, goat cheese, and radishes on top.
- Sprinkle the top lightly with a pinch of cinnamon. Set aside.

- In a small bowl, combine the olive oil together with the lemon juice, honey, and salt. Whisk to blend.
- Taste, and adjust the seasoning accordingly.
- Drizzle the dressing lightly over the salad.
- Serve and enjoy.

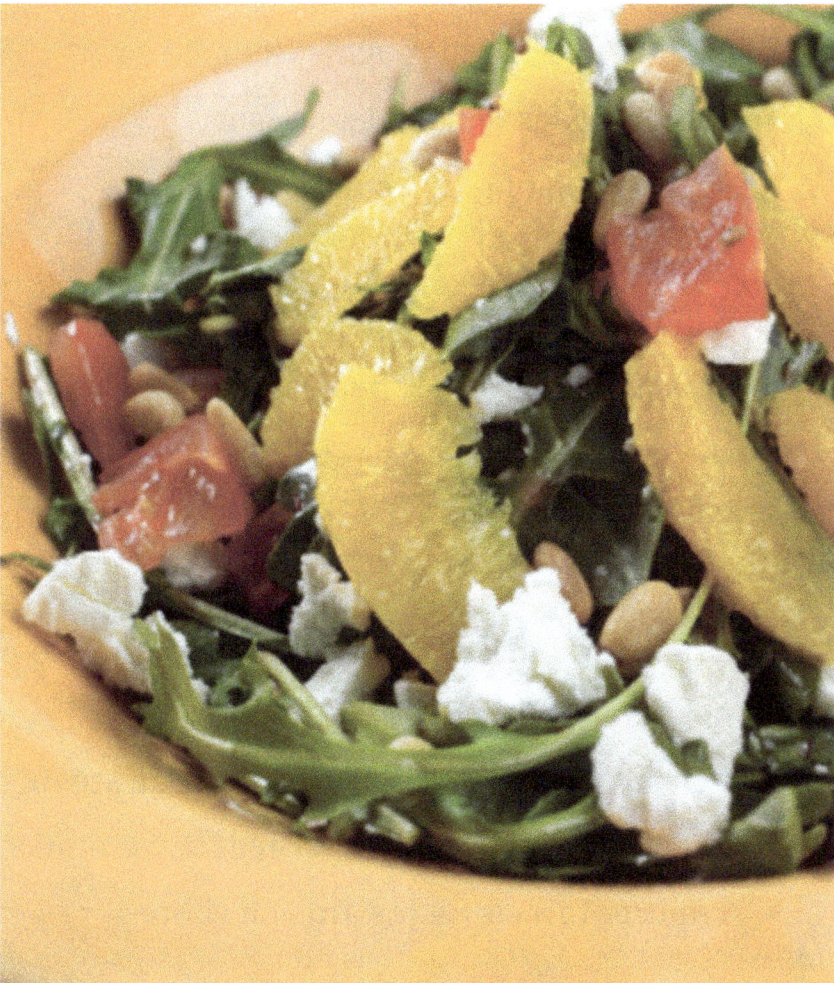

Celery salad with dates, almond, and parmesan

Ingredients

- ¼ cup of extra-virgin olive oil
- 2 ounces of Parmigiano-Reggiano cheese
- ½ cup of raw almonds
- 4 dates, pitted and roughly chopped
- 3 tablespoons of fresh lemon juice
- ¼ teaspoon of red pepper flakes
- Sea salt, to taste
- 8 long celery stalks
- Freshly ground black pepper, to taste

Directions

- Soak the celery in ice water for about 20 minutes.
- Drain and pat dry, then pile the celery into a medium serving bowl.
- Warm the almonds over medium heat, stirring often, until fragrant and toasted for 7 minutes.
- Transfer to a cutting board and chop.

- Add the celery leaves to the bowl of celery with chopped almonds, dates, lemon juice, and red pepper flakes.
- Season with salt and pepper, toss to combine.
- Add the cheese and olive oil, toss.
- Serve and enjoy.

Greek wedge salad

The Greek wedge salad takes pride in pilled vegetables on top mainly romaine lettuce, tomatoes, and olives. This Mediterranean Sea diet is best consumed immediately than later.

Ingredients

- 2 tablespoons of tahini
- 1 ½ cups of cherry tomatoes
- 3 cloves of garlic, minced
- ⅔ cup of cucumber
- ⅔ cup of chopped celery
- ¼ cup of pitted Kalamata olives
- Freshly ground black pepper
- 1 shallot, thinly sliced
- 2 heads of romaine
- ½ teaspoon of grain sea salt
- 1 tablespoon of lemon juice
- Pinch of salt
- ¼ cup of extra virgin olive oil
- 3 tablespoons of lemon juice

Directions

- In a medium mixing bowl, combine the tomatoes together with the cucumber, olives, shallot, lemon juice, celery, and a pinch of salt. Toss, let marinate.
- In a small bowl, combine extra virgin olive oil, lemon juice, tahini, garlic, sea salt, and black pepper, whisk.
- Season generously with pepper, whisk.
- Place each romaine halve on its own dinner plate.
- Top with the tomato salad mixture.
- Drizzle the dressing over the salads
- Serve and enjoy.

Massaged broccoli rabe salad with sunflower seeds and cranberries

This recipe turns broccoli to a delicious salad after dressing with garlicky and lemony and other herbs and seeds.

Ingredients

- 1 large clove garlic
- 2 bunches of broccoli rabe
- 1 tablespoon of lemon juice
- ¼ cup of sunflower seeds
- ½ teaspoon of Dijon mustard
- ½ cup of chopped celery
- ¼ teaspoon of salt
- ⅓ cup of grated Parmesan cheese
- ¼ cup of dried cranberries
- 3 tablespoons of olive oil

Directions

- In a medium skillet over medium heat, toast the sunflower seeds for 5 minutes.
- Remove, and set aside.

- In a small bowl, whisk together the lemon juice, mustard, olive oil, garlic, and salt until emulsified.
- Pour the dressing over the leaves and gently massage the dressing into the leaves.
- Taste, and adjust the seasoning.
- Add the chopped celery together with the grated Parmesan, toasted sunflower seeds, and dried cranberries to the serving bowl.
- Serve and enjoy.